WOMEN HEART SOLUTION

A Tried-and-True Programmed To Prevent and Treat Heart Disease In Women

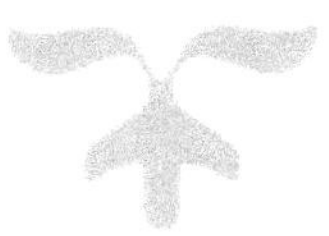

OLIVIA JONES

2 |WOMEN'S HEART SOLUTION

3 |WOMEN'S HEART SOLUTION

INTRODUCTION

Understanding Women's Heart Health

Heart disease is often considered a condition that primarily affects men. However, the reality is that it is the leading cause of death for women worldwide. Despite this alarming statistic, there remains a significant gap in understanding and awareness of heart disease in women. In this introduction, we will delve into the unique aspects of heart disease in women, emphasizing the importance of early detection and prevention.

The Unique Aspects of Heart Disease in Women

Historically, heart disease has been predominantly studied in men, leading to misconceptions that it primarily affects males. However, research has shown that women experience heart disease differently, often presenting with distinct symptoms and risk factors.

One of the key differences is the prevalence of coronary microvascular disease (CMD) in women. Unlike traditional coronary artery disease (CAD), which involves blockages in the major arteries supplying the heart, CMD affects the smaller blood vessels in the heart. This condition can lead to symptoms such as chest pain, shortness of breath, and fatigue, often without any significant blockages seen on standard diagnostic tests like angiograms.

Additionally, women are more likely to experience what are often referred to as "atypical" symptoms of heart disease. While chest pain is a common symptom for both men and women, women may also present with symptoms such as nausea, indigestion, jaw pain, or back pain. These symptoms are not always recognized as indicative of heart problems, leading to delays in diagnosis and treatment.

The Story of Elizabeth: A Personal Journey with Heart Disease

To illustrate the importance of understanding women's heart health, let us consider the story of Elizabeth, a vibrant and active woman in her early fifties. Elizabeth had always been conscientious about her health, maintaining a balanced diet and exercising regularly. However, she began experiencing occasional episodes of fatigue and discomfort in her chest during her daily walks.

Initially, Elizabeth dismissed these symptoms, attributing them to stress or overexertion. However, when the episodes became more frequent and intense, she decided to seek medical attention. After undergoing a series of tests, including a stress test and cardiac catheterization, Elizabeth was diagnosed with coronary microvascular disease (CMD). Despite having no significant blockages in her major coronary arteries, the small vessels in her heart were not functioning properly, leading to inadequate blood flow and symptoms of angina.

Elizabeth's story highlights the importance of recognizing the diverse ways in which heart disease can manifest in women. Despite her healthy lifestyle and absence of traditional risk factors such as smoking or obesity, she still developed a form of heart disease that is often overlooked in clinical settings.

Importance of Early Detection and Prevention

Early detection of heart disease is crucial for both men and women, but it is especially vital for women due to the unique nature of their symptoms and risk factors. Unfortunately, studies have shown that women are less likely than men to receive timely and appropriate care for heart-related issues, leading to worse outcomes.

Prevention is equally important, if not more so, in addressing the burden of heart disease in women.

Adopting a heart-healthy lifestyle that includes regular exercise, a balanced diet, stress management, and avoidance of tobacco is essential for reducing the risk of developing heart disease.

In conclusion, understanding the unique aspects of heart disease in women is paramount for early detection and prevention. By raising awareness, promoting education, and advocating for gender-sensitive healthcare practices, we can strive to improve outcomes and quality of life for women affected by heart disease.

This introduction sets the stage for the rest of the book, emphasizing the importance of understanding women's heart health and the need for early detection and prevention. Through the story of Elizabeth and an exploration of the unique aspects of heart disease in women, readers are encouraged to approach the topic with heightened awareness and diligence.

CHAPTER 2

Know Your Heart: Anatomy and Function

In this chapter, we will explore the intricate structure and vital functions of the female heart. Understanding the anatomy and physiology of the heart lays the foundation for comprehending its vulnerabilities and responses to various stimuli. Additionally, we will delve into the influence of hormones on heart health, considering their nuanced effects on the cardiovascular system.

Exploring the Structure and Function of the Female Heart

Anatomy of the Heart

The heart is a remarkable organ composed of four chambers: two atria and two ventricles. These chambers work in concert to pump blood throughout the body, delivering essential nutrients and oxygen while removing waste products. In women, the size and shape of the heart may differ slightly from that of men, influenced by factors such as body size and hormonal fluctuations.

The walls of the heart are comprised of specialized muscle tissue known as myocardium, which contracts rhythmically to propel blood forward. Surrounding the myocardium is a protective sac called the pericardium, which helps maintain the heart's position within the chest cavity and prevents friction during movement.

Circulation of Blood

The heart functions as a dual pump, with the right side responsible for pumping oxygen-depleted blood to the lungs for oxygenation, while the left side pumps oxygen-rich blood to the rest of the body. This process, known as systemic and pulmonary circulation, ensures a continuous supply of oxygenated blood to all tissues and organs.

The coronary arteries, which originate from the aorta, supply the heart muscle with oxygen and nutrients necessary for its function. Any disruption in coronary blood flow can lead to ischemia (lack of blood flow) and subsequent damage to the heart muscle, known as a heart attack or myocardial infarction.

Electrical Conduction System

The heartbeat is regulated by a complex network of specialized cells that generate and transmit electrical impulses throughout the heart. This electrical conduction system coordinates the rhythmic contraction of the atria and ventricles, ensuring efficient pumping action. Disruptions in the conduction system can result in arrhythmias, abnormal heart rhythms that may impair cardiac function.

How Hormones Influence Heart Health

Estrogen and Progesterone

Estrogen and progesterone, two primary female sex hormones, exert significant influence on heart health. Estrogen, in particular, has been shown to have cardio protective effects, including the promotion of vasodilation (widening of blood vessels), reduction of LDL cholesterol levels (the "bad" cholesterol), and inhibition of plaque formation in the arteries.

During reproductive years, estrogen levels fluctuate throughout the menstrual cycle, with peak levels occurring during the follicular phase. This cyclic variation in hormone levels may contribute to fluctuations in cardiovascular function, including changes in blood pressure and vascular tone.

Menopause and Hormonal Changes

The transition to menopause marks a significant hormonal shift in women, characterized by a decline in estrogen production and fluctuations in other hormones. This hormonal imbalance has been associated with an increased risk of cardiovascular disease, as estrogen's cardioprotective effects diminish.

Postmenopausal women are at higher risk of developing conditions such as hypertension, dyslipidemia (abnormal lipid levels), and metabolic syndrome, all of which contribute to the development of atherosclerosis and coronary artery disease.

Hormone Replacement Therapy (HRT)

Hormone replacement therapy (HRT) has been proposed as a potential strategy to mitigate the adverse effects of menopause on heart health. By supplementing estrogen and progesterone, HRT aims to restore hormonal balance and alleviate menopausal symptoms.

However, the use of HRT remains controversial due to conflicting evidence regarding its cardiovascular benefits and risks. While some studies suggest a reduction in cardiovascular events with HRT use, others have raised concerns about an increased risk of thromboembolic events (blood clots) and stroke.

We have explored the intricate anatomy and vital functions of the female heart, highlighting its unique characteristics and vulnerabilities. Additionally, we have examined the complex interplay between hormones and heart health, underscoring the importance of hormonal balance in maintaining cardiovascular well-being.

By understanding the structure, function, and hormonal regulation of the heart, women can take proactive steps to optimize their cardiovascular health and reduce their risk of heart disease. In the subsequent chapters, we will delve further into risk factors, prevention strategies, and treatment options specific to women's heart health, empowering readers to prioritize their cardiovascular well-being.

This detailed exploration of the female heart's anatomy, function, and hormonal influences provides readers with a comprehensive understanding of the factors that contribute to women's heart health. By elucidating the complexities of cardiac physiology and the intricate interplay of hormones, readers are equipped with valuable knowledge to make informed decisions regarding their cardiovascular well-being.

CHAPTER 3

Risk Factors for Heart Disease in Women

Heart disease is a significant health concern for women, and understanding the risk factors is crucial for prevention and early intervention. In this chapter, we will explore both traditional risk factors and gender-specific risk factors that contribute to heart disease in women. By identifying and managing these risk factors, women can take proactive steps to protect their heart health and reduce their risk of cardiovascular disease.

Identifying and Managing Traditional Risk Factors

1. High Blood Pressure (Hypertension)

High blood pressure, or hypertension, is a leading risk factor for heart disease in women. It places increased strain on the heart and blood vessels, leading to damage over time. Hypertension often goes unnoticed as it typically presents with no symptoms, earning it the nickname "the silent killer."

Managing blood pressure involves lifestyle modifications such as adopting a heart-healthy diet low in sodium and saturated fats, engaging in regular physical activity, maintaining a healthy weight, limiting alcohol intake, and managing stress. In some cases, medication may be necessary to control blood pressure levels effectively.

2. High Cholesterol (Dyslipidemia)

Elevated levels of cholesterol, particularly low-density lipoprotein (LDL) cholesterol, contribute to the buildup of plaque in the arteries, leading to atherosclerosis and an increased risk of heart disease. Additionally, low levels of high-density lipoprotein (HDL) cholesterol, known as "good" cholesterol, can also be a risk factor for heart disease.

Managing cholesterol levels involves adopting a heart-healthy diet rich in fruits, vegetables, whole grains, and lean proteins, as well as avoiding trans fats and saturated fats. Regular exercise and maintaining a healthy weight can also help lower cholesterol levels. In some cases, medication, such as statins, may be prescribed to effectively manage cholesterol levels.

3. Diabetes Mellitus

Diabetes mellitus, particularly type 2 diabetes, significantly increases the risk of heart disease in women. Elevated blood sugar levels can damage blood vessels and nerves over time, increasing the likelihood of developing cardiovascular complications such as coronary artery disease, heart attack, and stroke.

Managing diabetes involves maintaining tight control of blood sugar levels through a combination of medication, insulin therapy (if necessary), regular monitoring of blood glucose levels, adopting a healthy diet, engaging in regular physical activity, and maintaining a healthy weight. It is essential for women with diabetes to work closely with their healthcare providers to develop a comprehensive management plan tailored to their individual needs.

Recognizing Gender-Specific Risk Factors

1. Hormonal Changes

Hormonal fluctuations throughout a woman's life can influence her risk of heart disease. Estrogen, a female sex hormone, has been shown to have cardio protective effects, including the promotion of vasodilation, reduction of LDL cholesterol levels, and inhibition of plaque formation in the arteries. However, during menopause, estrogen levels decline, increasing a woman's risk of developing heart disease.

Additionally, certain hormonal conditions such as polycystic ovary syndrome (PCOS) and pregnancy-related conditions like gestational diabetes and preeclampsia can increase the risk of heart disease in women. It is essential for women to be aware of these hormonal changes and discuss any concerns with their healthcare providers.

2. Pregnancy Complications

Complications during pregnancy, such as gestational diabetes and preeclampsia, can increase a woman's risk of developing heart disease later in life. Gestational diabetes, characterized by elevated blood sugar levels during pregnancy, is associated with an increased risk of developing type 2 diabetes and heart disease in the future.

Preeclampsia, a condition characterized by high blood pressure and protein in the urine during pregnancy, can also increase the risk of developing hypertension and heart disease later in life. Women who have experienced complications during pregnancy should be vigilant about monitoring their heart health and discussing any concerns with their healthcare providers.

3. Autoimmune Diseases

Autoimmune diseases, such as rheumatoid arthritis, lupus, and psoriasis, are more common in women and have been associated with an increased risk of heart disease. These conditions can cause inflammation in the body, including the arteries, leading to atherosclerosis and an increased risk of heart attack and stroke.

Managing autoimmune diseases involves working closely with healthcare providers to control symptoms and reduce inflammation. Adopting a healthy lifestyle, including regular exercise, maintaining a healthy weight, and avoiding smoking, can also help reduce the risk of heart disease in women with autoimmune conditions.

Understanding both traditional risk factors and gender-specific risk factors is essential for protecting women's heart health. By identifying and managing these risk factors, women can take proactive steps to their risk of heart disease and live longer, healthier lives. In the subsequent chapters, we will explore prevention strategies and treatment options specific to women's heart health, empowering readers to prioritize their cardiovascular well-being.

This comprehensive reduce exploration of traditional and gender-specific risk factors for heart disease in women highlights the importance of awareness and proactive management. By recognizing and addressing these risk factors, women can take control of their heart health and reduce their risk of cardiovascular disease. Through lifestyle modifications, close monitoring, and collaboration with healthcare providers, women can optimize their cardiovascular well-being and enjoy a higher quality of life.

CHAPTER 4

Healthy Lifestyle Habits for a Strong Heart

Maintaining a healthy lifestyle is crucial for promoting heart health and reducing the risk of cardiovascular disease. In this chapter, we will explore four essential lifestyle habits that can support a strong and resilient heart: nutrition guidelines for heart health, the role of exercise in preventing heart disease, stress management techniques, and the importance of adequate sleep.

Nutrition Guidelines for Heart Health

1. Eat a Balanced Diet

A heart-healthy diet emphasizes whole, nutrient-rich foods while minimizing processed and refined foods high in added sugars, unhealthy fats, and sodium. Key components of a heart-healthy diet include:

Fruits and vegetables: Aim to include a variety of colorful fruits and vegetables in your diet, as they are rich in vitamins, minerals, antioxidants, and dietary fiber, which can help lower blood pressure and reduce the risk of heart disease.

Whole grains: Choose whole grains such as brown rice, quinoa, oats, and whole wheat bread, which are rich in fiber and nutrients and can help lower cholesterol levels and improve heart health.

Lean proteins: Opt for lean sources of protein such as poultry, fish, beans, legumes, tofu, and nuts, which are lower in saturated fats and cholesterol compared to red and processed meats.

Healthy fats: Include sources of healthy fats such as avocados, nuts, seeds, and olive oil, which can help improve cholesterol levels and reduce the risk of heart disease. Limit saturated and trans fats found in fried foods, baked goods, and processed snacks.

2. Watch Your Portions

Portion control is key to maintaining a healthy weight and preventing overeating, which can contribute to weight gain and obesity, both of which are risk factors for heart disease. Pay attention to serving sizes and try to eat mindfully, savoring each bite and stopping when you feel satisfied rather than overly full.

3. Limit Sodium Intake

Excessive sodium intake can increase blood pressure and strain the heart, increasing the risk of heart disease and stroke. Aim to limit sodium intake by choosing low-sodium or sodium-free options when possible, cooking at home using fresh ingredients, and avoiding processed and packaged foods high in sodium.

4. Stay Hydrated

Drinking an adequate amount of water is essential for heart health and overall well-being. Aim to drink plenty of water throughout the day and limit intake of sugary beverages such as soda, sports drinks, and fruit juices, which can contribute to weight gain and increase the risk of heart disease.

The Role of Exercise in Preventing Heart Disease

1. Aerobic Exercise

Regular aerobic exercise, such as brisk walking, jogging, cycling, swimming, or dancing, is essential for maintaining cardiovascular health and reducing the risk of heart disease. Aerobic exercise helps strengthen the heart muscle, improve circulation, lower blood pressure, and reduce LDL cholesterol levels, all of which contribute to a healthier heart.

2. Strength Training

In addition to aerobic exercise, strength training is also beneficial for heart health. Strength training exercises, such as lifting weights, using resistance bands, or performing bodyweight exercises, help build and maintain muscle mass, improve metabolism, and promote overall physical fitness.

3. Flexibility and Balance Exercises

Incorporating flexibility and balance exercises into your routine can help improve mobility, reduce the risk of injury, and enhance overall physical well-being. Activities such as yoga, tai chi, and Pilates can improve flexibility, balance, and coordination while promoting relaxation and stress reduction.

4. Aim for Consistency and Variety

To reap the full benefits of exercise, it's important to be consistent with your workouts and vary your routine to prevent boredom and plateauing. Aim for at least 150 minutes of moderate-intensity aerobic exercise or 75 minutes of vigorous-intensity aerobic exercise per week, along with two or more days of strength training exercises targeting major muscle groups.

Adopting healthy lifestyle habits, including following nutrition guidelines for heart health and incorporating regular exercise into your routine, is essential for maintaining a strong and resilient heart. By making small, sustainable changes to your diet and exercise habits, you can reduce your risk of heart disease and improve your overall health and well-being. In the subsequent chapters, we will explore additional strategies for promoting heart health, including stress management techniques and the importance of adequate sleep.

This detailed exploration of nutrition guidelines for heart health and the role of exercise in preventing heart disease provides readers with practical strategies for maintaining a strong and resilient heart. By incorporating these healthy lifestyle habits into their daily routine, readers can optimize their cardiovascular health and reduce their risk of heart disease. Through mindful eating, regular physical activity, and consistency in exercise, individuals can take proactive steps to protect their heart health and improve their overall well-being.

CHAPTER 5

Stress Management and Heart Health

Stress is a natural response to life's challenges, but chronic or excessive stress can have detrimental effects on heart health. In this chapter, we will explore the connection between stress and heart disease, as well as strategies for coping and relaxation to promote heart health and overall well-being.

Understanding the Connection Between Stress and Heart Disease

1. The Stress Response

When faced with a stressful situation, the body's natural response is to release hormones such as adrenaline and cortisol, which prepare the body for "fight or flight." While this response is necessary for survival in acute situations, chronic stress can lead to persistent activation of the stress response system, resulting in long-term physiological and psychological consequences.

2. Impact of Chronic Stress on Heart Health

Chronic stress has been linked to an increased risk of heart disease and other cardiovascular conditions. Prolonged exposure to stress hormones can lead to elevated blood pressure, increased heart rate, inflammation, and changes in blood clotting, all of which can contribute to the development of atherosclerosis, heart attack, and stroke.

3. Psychological Factors

In addition to physiological changes, psychological factors such as depression, anxiety, and social isolation can also contribute to the link between stress and heart disease. People experiencing chronic stress may engage in unhealthy coping mechanisms such as smoking, overeating, or excessive alcohol consumption, further increasing their risk of heart disease.

Strategies for Coping and Relaxation

1. Mindfulness and Meditation

Mindfulness and meditation practices can help reduce stress and promote relaxation by fostering present-moment awareness and acceptance. Mindfulness techniques such as deep breathing, body scan meditation, and mindfulness-based stress reduction (MBSR) have been shown to lower blood pressure, reduce anxiety, and improve overall well-being.

2. Exercise

Regular physical activity is not only beneficial for heart health but also serves as a powerful stress management tool. Exercise helps release endorphins, the body's natural mood-boosting hormones, and provides a healthy outlet for pent-up energy and tension. Aim for at least 30 minutes of moderate-intensity exercise most days of the week to reap the stress-relieving benefits.

3. Relaxation Techniques

Incorporating relaxation techniques into your daily routine can help counteract the effects of stress and promote a sense of calm and well-being. Techniques such as progressive muscle relaxation, guided imagery, and visualization can help relax the body and quiet the mind, reducing muscle tension and promoting a state of relaxation.

4. Social Support

Maintaining strong social connections and seeking support from friends, family, or support groups can help buffer the effects of stress and promote resilience. Having a supportive network of people to lean on during challenging times can provide emotional validation, practical assistance, and a sense of belonging, all of which are essential for coping with stress.

5. Healthy Lifestyle Habits

Adopting healthy lifestyle habits such as eating a balanced diet, getting regular exercise, prioritizing sleep, and avoiding excessive alcohol and caffeine can help support overall well-being and resilience to stress. Nourishing your body with nutrient-rich foods, staying physically active, and getting adequate rest are essential for maintaining a strong and resilient body and mind.

Managing stress is essential for maintaining heart health and overall well-being. By understanding the connection between stress and heart disease and adopting effective coping strategies and relaxation techniques, individuals can reduce their risk of cardiovascular disease and improve their quality of life. In the subsequent chapters, we will explore additional strategies for promoting heart health, including the importance of adequate sleep and the benefits of positive lifestyle habits.

This comprehensive exploration of stress management and heart health provides readers with practical strategies for coping with stress and promoting relaxation. By incorporating mindfulness, exercise, relaxation techniques, social support, and healthy lifestyle habits into their daily routine, individuals can reduce their risk of heart disease and improve their overall well-being. Through proactive stress management, individuals can protect their heart health and enjoy a higher quality of life.

CHAPTER 6

Understanding Heart Disease Symptoms in Women

Recognizing the signs and symptoms of heart disease is crucial for early detection and prompt treatment, particularly in women who may experience atypical or subtle symptoms. In this chapter, we will explore the unique presentation of heart disease symptoms in women, highlighting atypical signs and symptoms and emphasizing the importance of seeking prompt medical attention.

Recognizing Atypical Signs and Symptoms

1. Chest Pain or Discomfort

While chest pain is a common symptom of heart disease in both men and women, women may experience atypical chest pain that differs from the classic "crushing" or "pressure-like" sensation often described by men. Women may experience chest discomfort that feels more like tightness, squeezing, fullness, or burning rather than pain. Additionally, chest pain in women may be more diffuse and radiate to other areas of the body such as the back, neck, jaw, shoulders, or arms.

2. Shortness of Breath

Shortness of breath, or dyspnea, is another common symptom of heart disease in women. Women may experience difficulty breathing or feel breathless even during minimal exertion or at rest. Shortness of breath may be accompanied by other symptoms such as chest discomfort, fatigue, dizziness, or palpitations.

3. Fatigue

Unexplained fatigue or extreme tiredness is a common symptom of heart disease in women. Women may experience fatigue that is not relieved by rest and interferes with daily activities. Fatigue may be accompanied by other symptoms such as chest discomfort, shortness of breath, nausea, or lightheadedness.

4. Nausea or Indigestion

Nausea, vomiting, or indigestion may be atypical symptoms of heart disease in women. Women may mistake these symptoms for gastrointestinal issues or food poisoning, leading to delays in seeking medical attention. Nausea or indigestion may be accompanied by other symptoms such as chest discomfort, shortness of breath, or fatigue.

5. Dizziness or Lightheadedness

Dizziness, lightheadedness, or fainting spells may be warning signs of heart disease in women. Women may experience feelings of lightheadedness or dizziness, particularly when standing up quickly or exerting themselves. These symptoms may be accompanied by other signs such as chest discomfort, shortness of breath, or palpitations.

6. Palpitations

Heart palpitations, or sensations of irregular or rapid heartbeat, may be a symptom of heart disease in women. Women may experience palpitations that feel like fluttering, pounding, or racing sensations in the chest. Palpitations may occur at rest or during physical activity and may be accompanied by other symptoms such as chest discomfort, shortness of breath, or dizziness.

Seeking Prompt Medical Attention

1. Know Your Risk Factors

Understanding your risk factors for heart disease is essential for early detection and prevention. Women with risk factors such as high blood pressure, high cholesterol, diabetes, obesity, smoking, or a family history of heart disease should be particularly vigilant about monitoring their heart health and seeking medical attention if they experience any symptoms of concern.

2. Trust Your Instincts

If you experience symptoms that are unusual or concerning, trust your instincts and seek medical attention promptly. Women often downplay or dismiss their symptoms, attributing them to stress, anxiety, or other benign causes. However, it is essential to take any symptoms of heart disease seriously and seek evaluation by a healthcare professional.

3. Act Quickly

Time is of the essence when it comes to heart disease, as prompt treatment can make a significant difference in outcomes. If you experience symptoms such as chest discomfort, shortness of breath, fatigue, nausea, dizziness, or palpitations, do not hesitate to call emergency services or go to the nearest emergency department for evaluation and treatment.

4. Be Your Own Advocate

Women are often underdiagnosed and undertreated for heart disease, as their symptoms may be overlooked or attributed to other causes. Be your own advocate and insist on a thorough evaluation if you suspect you may be experiencing symptoms of heart disease. Ask questions, seek second opinions if necessary, and advocate for the care you deserve

Understanding the signs and symptoms of heart disease in women is essential for early detection and prompt treatment. By recognizing atypical signs and symptoms and seeking prompt medical attention, women can reduce their risk of complications and improve their outcomes. In the subsequent chapters, we will explore diagnostic tests and screening methods for heart disease, empowering women to take charge of their heart health and well-being.

This comprehensive exploration of understanding heart disease symptoms in women provides readers with valuable insights into recognizing atypical signs and symptoms and the importance of seeking prompt medical attention. By understanding the unique presentation of heart disease symptoms in women and taking proactive steps to seek evaluation and treatment, individuals can protect their heart health and improve their outcomes. Through awareness, advocacy, and timely intervention, women can prioritize their cardiovascular well-being and enjoy a higher quality of life.

CHAPTER 7

Diagnostic Tests and Screening

Diagnostic tests and screening play a crucial role in identifying heart disease and assessing cardiovascular risk. In this chapter, we will provide an overview of common diagnostic tests for heart disease, discuss the importance of regular screening for women, and empower individuals to take proactive steps in protecting their heart health.

Overview of Common Tests for Heart Disease

1. Electrocardiogram (ECG or EKG)

An electrocardiogram is a non-invasive test that measures the electrical activity of the heart. It can detect abnormal heart rhythms, ischemia (lack of blood flow to the heart muscle), and other cardiac abnormalities. During an ECG, electrodes are placed on the chest, arms, and legs, and the electrical signals produced by the heart are recorded and analyzed by a healthcare provider.

2. Echocardiogram

An echocardiogram is a non-invasive test that uses sound waves to create images of the heart's structure and function. It can assess the size and shape of the heart, the function of the heart valves, and the movement of the heart muscle. Echocardiography is useful for diagnosing conditions such as heart failure, valve disorders, and congenital heart defects.

3. Stress Test

A stress test, also known as an exercise stress test or treadmill test, evaluates the heart's response to physical activity. During a stress test, the patient exercises on a treadmill or stationary bike while their heart rate, blood pressure, and ECG are monitored. Stress testing can help diagnose coronary artery disease, assess exercise tolerance, and evaluate the effectiveness of treatment.

4. Coronary Angiography

Coronary angiography is an invasive test that uses X-ray imaging to visualize the coronary arteries. A special dye is injected into the arteries, allowing healthcare providers to identify blockages or narrowing in the arteries that supply blood to the heart muscle. Coronary angiography is commonly used to diagnose coronary artery disease and determine the need for interventions such as angioplasty or stenting.

5. Cardiac CT or MRI

Cardiac computed tomography (CT) and magnetic resonance imaging (MRI) are non-invasive imaging tests that provide detailed images of the heart and blood vessels. These tests can assess the structure and function of the heart, detect abnormalities such as tumors or blood clots, and evaluate blood flow in the coronary arteries. Cardiac CT and MRI are useful for diagnosing a wide range of heart conditions and guiding treatment decisions.

Importance of Regular Screening for Women

1. Heart Disease Risk in Women

Heart disease is the leading cause of death among women worldwide, yet it is often underdiagnosed and undertreated in women compared to men. Women may present with atypical symptoms or delay seeking medical attention, leading to delays in diagnosis and treatment. Regular screening can help identify heart disease early and facilitate timely intervention.

2. Unique Risk Factors in Women

Women may have unique risk factors for heart disease, including hormonal changes associated with menopause, pregnancy-related conditions such as gestational diabetes and preeclampsia, and autoimmune diseases such as rheumatoid arthritis and lupus. Regular screening can help identify these risk factors and allow for early intervention to reduce the risk of heart disease.

3. Preventive Care and Risk Assessment

Regular screening allows healthcare providers to assess an individual's risk of heart disease and develop personalized preventive care plans. Screening tests such as blood pressure measurement, cholesterol screening, and diabetes testing can help identify modifiable risk factors and guide lifestyle modifications and treatment decisions to reduce the risk of heart disease.

4. Empowerment and Advocacy

Regular screening empowers women to take charge of their heart health and advocate for their well-being. By proactively seeking preventive care and participating in screening tests, women can prioritize their cardiovascular health and reduce their risk of heart disease. Screening also provides an opportunity for education and awareness about heart disease risk factors and prevention strategies.

Regular screening and diagnostic testing are essential components of preventive care for heart disease in women. By undergoing routine screening tests and diagnostic evaluations, women can identify heart disease early, assess their risk factors, and take proactive steps to protect their heart health. Through awareness, education, and advocacy, women can prioritize their cardiovascular well-being and enjoy a higher quality of life.

This comprehensive overview of diagnostic tests and screening for heart disease underscores the importance of regular screening for women. By understanding the role of diagnostic tests in identifying heart disease and assessing cardiovascular risk, women can take proactive steps to protect their heart health and reduce their risk of heart disease-related complications. Through empowerment, education, and advocacy, women can prioritize their cardiovascular well-being and enjoy a higher quality of life.

CHAPTER 8

Treatment Options for Women with Heart Disease

Effective treatment of heart disease in women involves a multifaceted approach that may include medications, procedures, and surgeries tailored to individual needs. In this chapter, we will explore various treatment options available for women with heart disease, empowering them to make informed decisions about their care and improve their cardiovascular health and well-being.

Medications

1. Statins

Statins are medications that lower cholesterol levels by inhibiting the enzyme responsible for cholesterol production in the liver. They are commonly prescribed to reduce LDL cholesterol levels and lower the risk of cardiovascular events such as heart attack and stroke. Statins may also have anti-inflammatory effects that benefit overall cardiovascular health.

2. ACE Inhibitors and ARBs

Angiotensin-converting enzyme (ACE) inhibitors and angiotensin II receptor blockers (ARBs) are medications that help lower blood pressure and reduce strain on the heart. They are commonly prescribed to treat high blood pressure, heart failure, and other cardiovascular conditions. ACE inhibitors and ARBs can help improve heart function and reduce the risk of complications in women with heart disease.

3. Beta-Blockers

Beta-blockers are medications that block the effects of adrenaline on the heart, reducing heart rate and blood pressure. They are commonly prescribed to treat high blood pressure, angina (chest pain), heart failure, and arrhythmias (irregular heart rhythms). Beta-blockers can help improve symptoms and reduce the risk of cardiovascular events in women with heart disease.

4. Antiplatelet Agents

Antiplatelet agents such as aspirin and clopidogrel help prevent blood clot formation by inhibiting platelet aggregation. They are commonly prescribed to reduce the risk of blood clots and cardiovascular events such as heart attack and stroke. Antiplatelet therapy is often recommended for women with a history of heart attack, stroke, or certain cardiovascular conditions.

5. Anticoagulants

Anticoagulants, or blood thinners, help prevent blood clot formation and reduce the risk of stroke and other thrombotic events. They are commonly prescribed to treat conditions such as atrial fibrillation, deep vein thrombosis, and pulmonary embolism. Anticoagulant therapy may be recommended for women with certain cardiovascular conditions or risk factors for thrombosis.

Procedures

1. Angioplasty and Stenting

Angioplasty, also known as percutaneous coronary intervention (PCI), is a minimally invasive procedure used to open blocked or narrowed coronary arteries. During angioplasty, a catheter with a balloon at the tip is inserted into the blocked artery and inflated to widen the artery and improve blood flow. In some cases, a stent (a small mesh tube) may be placed in the artery to help keep it open.

2. Coronary Artery Bypass Grafting (CABG)

Coronary artery bypass grafting (CABG) is a surgical procedure used to bypass blocked or narrowed coronary arteries. During CABG, a healthy blood vessel from another part of the body is harvested and attached to the coronary artery to create a new pathway for blood flow. CABG is typically reserved for women with severe coronary artery disease who have not responded to other treatments.

3. Heart Valve Repair or Replacement

Heart valve repair or replacement may be necessary for women with heart valve disease, such as aortic stenosis or mitral regurgitation. Valve repair involves surgical repair of the damaged valve, while valve replacement involves replacing the damaged valve with a mechanical or biological valve. Valve repair or replacement can improve symptoms and quality of life in women with heart valve disease.

4. Pacemaker or Implantable Cardioverter-Defibrillator (ICD)

A pacemaker or implantable cardioverter-defibrillator (ICD) may be recommended for women with certain arrhythmias or heart rhythm disorders. A pacemaker is a small device that helps regulate the heart's rhythm by delivering electrical impulses to the heart muscle. An ICD is a device that monitors the heart rhythm and delivers a shock to restore normal rhythm if a life-threatening arrhythmia occurs.

Tailoring Treatment Plans to Individual Needs

1. Personalized Approach

Treatment of heart disease in women should be tailored to individual needs, taking into account factors such as age, overall health, underlying conditions, and preferences. Healthcare providers should work closely with women to develop personalized treatment plans that address their unique needs and goals.

2. Shared Decision Making

Shared decision making involves collaboration between healthcare providers and patients in making treatment decisions. Women should be actively involved in decisions about their care, including discussions about treatment options, risks and benefits, and preferences. Shared decision making empowers women to make informed choices about their health and well-being.

3. Comprehensive Care

Comprehensive care for heart disease in women involves addressing not only the physical aspects of the condition but also the emotional, social, and psychological aspects. Women should have access to a multidisciplinary team of healthcare providers, including cardiologists, nurses, dietitians, physical therapists, and mental health professionals, to provide comprehensive care and support.

4. Lifestyle Modification

Lifestyle modification is an essential component of treatment for heart disease in women. Women should be encouraged to adopt heart-healthy habits such as eating a balanced diet, engaging in regular physical activity, maintaining a healthy weight, quitting smoking, and managing stress. Lifestyle modification can help improve cardiovascular health and reduce the risk of complications.

Treatment of heart disease in women involves a comprehensive approach that may include medications, procedures, and surgeries tailored to individual needs. By understanding the various treatment options available and actively participating in decision making about their care, women can take control of their heart health and improve their outcomes. Through personalized treatment plans, comprehensive care, and lifestyle modification, women can optimize their cardiovascular health and enjoy a higher quality of life.

This comprehensive exploration of treatment options for women with heart disease provides readers with valuable insights into medications, procedures, and surgeries available to manage heart disease. By understanding the importance of tailoring treatment plans to individual needs and actively participating in decision making about their care, women can take proactive steps to protect their heart health and improve their outcomes. Through personalized treatment approaches, comprehensive care, and lifestyle modification, women can prioritize their cardiovascular well-being and enjoy a higher quality of life.

CHAPTER 9

Living Well with Heart Disease

Adjusting to life after a diagnosis of heart disease can be challenging, but with the right support systems and resources, women can thrive and maintain a high quality of life. In this chapter, we will explore strategies for living well with heart disease, including adjusting to life after diagnosis and accessing support systems and resources tailored to women's needs.

Adjusting to Life After Diagnosis

1. Acceptance and Acknowledgment

Adjusting to life after a diagnosis of heart disease begins with acceptance and acknowledgment of the diagnosis. It's normal to experience a range of emotions, including shock, fear, anger, and sadness, but acknowledging the diagnosis is the first step toward moving forward and taking control of your health.

2. Education and Empowerment

Education is key to living well with heart disease. Take the time to learn about your condition, treatment options, and lifestyle modifications that can improve your cardiovascular health. Empower yourself with knowledge and become an active participant in your care by asking questions, seeking information from reliable sources, and advocating for your needs.

3. Lifestyle Modifications

Making lifestyle modifications is essential for managing heart disease and improving outcomes. Adopt heart-healthy habits such as eating a balanced diet, engaging in regular physical activity, maintaining a healthy weight, quitting smoking, and managing stress. Small changes can have a big impact on your cardiovascular health and overall well-being.

4. Emotional Support

Seeking emotional support from friends, family, support groups, or mental health professionals can help you cope with the emotional challenges of living with heart disease. Share your feelings with trusted individuals, seek out peer support from others who have experienced similar challenges, and consider counseling or therapy if needed.

Support Systems and Resources for Women

1. Healthcare Providers

Establishing a relationship with a healthcare provider who specializes in women's heart health is essential for comprehensive care. Women-specific heart health clinics or programs may offer specialized services tailored to women's needs, including risk assessment, preventive care, and management of heart disease.

2. Support Groups

Joining a support group for women with heart disease can provide valuable emotional support, encouragement, and camaraderie. Support groups offer a safe space to share experiences, ask questions, and learn from others who have faced similar challenges. Online support groups can also be a convenient option for women who may not have access to in-person meetings.

3. Patient Education Programs

Patient education programs and resources provide valuable information and support for women living with heart disease. Look for educational materials, workshops, webinars, and online resources offered by reputable organizations such as the American Heart Association, Women Heart: The National Coalition for Women with Heart Disease, and the National Heart, Lung, and Blood Institute.

4. Lifestyle Coaching

Lifestyle coaching programs can help women make sustainable lifestyle changes to improve their

61 |WOMEN'S HEART SOLUTION

cardiovascular health. These programs may offer personalized coaching, goal setting, behavior change strategies, and ongoing support to help women adopt and maintain heart-healthy habits.

5. Cardiac Rehabilitation

Cardiac rehabilitation programs are comprehensive, multidisciplinary programs designed to help individuals recover from heart disease and improve their overall cardiovascular health. These programs typically include exercise training, education, counseling, and support to help women manage their condition and reduce the risk of future complications.

Living well with heart disease is possible with the right support systems and resources in place. By adjusting to life after diagnosis, making lifestyle modifications, seeking emotional support, and accessing support systems and resources tailored to women's needs, women can thrive and maintain a high quality of life despite their diagnosis. Through education, empowerment, and engagement with healthcare providers and support networks, women can take control of their heart health and live life to the fullest.

This comprehensive exploration of living well with heart disease provides readers with valuable insights into adjusting to life after diagnosis and accessing support systems and resources tailored to women's needs. By embracing education, empowerment, lifestyle modifications, and emotional support, women can navigate the challenges of living with heart disease and thrive in spite of their diagnosis. Through engagement with healthcare providers, support networks, and community resources, women can prioritize their cardiovascular well-being and enjoy a fulfilling and meaningful life.

CHAPTER 10

Heart-Healthy Eating Plans

Maintaining a heart-healthy diet is essential for managing heart disease and reducing the risk of cardiovascular complications. In this chapter, we will provide sample meal plans and recipes for heart-healthy eating, along with tips for dining out and grocery shopping to support optimal cardiovascular health.

Sample Meal Plans

Day 1

Breakfast:

Overnight oats made with rolled oats, almond milk, chia seeds, and sliced strawberries

A handful of almonds

Green tea

Lunch:

Quinoa salad with mixed greens, cherry tomatoes, cucumber, avocado, and grilled chicken breast, dressed with lemon vinaigrette

Apple slices with almond butter

Dinner:

Baked salmon with lemon and herbs

Steamed broccoli

Quinoa pilaf with spinach and pine nuts

Mixed berry salad with a drizzle of honey

Day 2

Breakfast:

Greek yogurt parfait with low-fat Greek yogurt, granola, and mixed berries

Whole grain toast with avocado

Lunch:

Lentil soup with vegetables

Mixed green salad with balsamic vinaigrette

Orange slices

Dinner:

Grilled tofu skewers with bell peppers, onions, and zucchini

Brown rice pilaf with peas and carrots

Steamed asparagus

Sliced mango for dessert

Day 3

Breakfast:

Spinach and feta omelet

Whole grain toast with almond butter

Orange juice

Lunch:

Quinoa and black bean salad with diced bell peppers, corn, tomatoes, and cilantro

Baby carrots with hummus

Baked chicken breast with rosemary and garlic

Roasted sweet potatoes

Steamed green beans

Mixed berry smoothie for dessert

Heart-Healthy Recipes

1. Baked Salmon with Lemon and Herbs

Ingredients:

4 salmon fillets

2 tablespoons olive oil

1 lemon, thinly sliced

2 cloves garlic, minced

1 teaspoon dried thyme

1 teaspoon dried oregano

Salt and pepper to taste

Instructions:

Preheat the oven to 375°F (190°C).

Place the salmon fillets on a baking sheet lined with parchment paper.

Drizzle the salmon with olive oil and sprinkle with minced garlic, dried thyme, dried oregano, salt, and pepper.

Arrange lemon slices on top of the salmon.

Bake in the preheated oven for 12-15 minutes, or until the salmon is cooked through and flakes easily with a fork.

2. Quinoa and Black Bean Salad

Ingredients:

1 cup cooked quinoa

1 can black beans, rinsed and drained

1 cup diced bell peppers (red, yellow, or orange)

1 cup corn kernels (fresh or frozen)

1 cup cherry tomatoes, halved

1/4 cup chopped fresh cilantro

Juice of 1 lime

2 tablespoons olive oil

Salt and pepper to taste

Instructions:

In a large mixing bowl, combine cooked quinoa, black beans, diced bell peppers, corn kernels, cherry tomatoes, and chopped cilantro.

In a small bowl, whisk together lime juice, olive oil, salt, and pepper.

Pour the dressing over the quinoa mixture and toss until well combined.

Serve chilled or at room temperature.

Tips for Dining Out and Grocery Shopping

Dining Out:

- Choose restaurants that offer heart-healthy options, such as grilled fish, lean protein, and vegetable-based dishes.

- Opt for baked, broiled, steamed, or grilled items instead of fried or heavily sauced dishes.

- Ask for dressings and sauces on the side, and use them sparingly.

- Watch portion sizes and consider sharing entrees or taking leftovers home.

- Be mindful of hidden sources of sodium and saturated fat, such as cheese, bacon, and creamy sauces.

- Grocery Shopping:

- Plan meals and snacks ahead of time and make a grocery list to avoid impulse purchases.

- Choose fresh, whole foods whenever possible, such as fruits, vegetables, whole grains, lean protein, and low-fat dairy products.

- Read food labels and choose products with lower sodium, saturated fat, and added sugars.

- Stock up on heart-healthy staples such as olive oil, nuts, seeds, beans, lentils, and whole grains.

- Shop the perimeter of the grocery store, where fresh produce, meats, and dairy products are typically located, and avoid the aisles with processed and packaged foods.

Maintaining a heart-healthy diet is essential for managing heart disease and reducing the risk of cardiovascular complications. By following sample meal plans and recipes, incorporating heart-healthy ingredients, and practicing mindful eating habits, individuals can support optimal cardiovascular health and improve their overall well-being. Through informed choices at the grocery store and when dining out, individuals can prioritize their heart health and enjoy a satisfying and nourishing diet that promotes longevity and vitality.

This comprehensive exploration of heart-healthy eating plans provides readers with valuable sample meal plans, recipes, and tips for dining out and grocery shopping. By incorporating heart-healthy ingredients, making informed choices, and practicing mindful eating habits, individuals can support optimal cardiovascular health and improve their overall well-being. Through planning, preparation, and a commitment to heart-healthy eating, individuals can enjoy delicious and nutritious meals that promote longevity and vitality.

CHAPTER 11

Empowering Women to Take Charge of Their Heart Health

Empowering women to take charge of their heart health is crucial for early detection, prevention, and effective management of heart disease. In this chapter, we will explore strategies for advocating for oneself in healthcare settings and spreading awareness and education in the community to promote women's heart health.

Advocating for Yourself in Healthcare Settings

1. Know Your Risk Factors

Understanding your risk factors for heart disease is essential for advocating for your health. Be aware of factors such as family history, high blood pressure, high cholesterol, diabetes, obesity, smoking, and sedentary lifestyle. Discuss your risk factors with your healthcare provider and work together to develop a personalized prevention plan.

2. Be Informed

Educate yourself about heart disease, its symptoms, risk factors, and treatment options. Stay informed about the latest research and guidelines for women's heart health. Ask questions, seek clarification, and advocate for yourself during medical appointments. Request explanations in plain language and seek second opinions if needed.

3. Be Proactive

Take a proactive approach to your health by scheduling regular check-ups, screenings, and preventive care appointments. Monitor your blood pressure, cholesterol levels, and other cardiovascular risk factors regularly. Keep track of your symptoms, medications, and lifestyle habits, and communicate any changes or concerns to your healthcare provider.

4. Engage in Shared Decision Making

Participate in shared decision making with your healthcare provider when discussing treatment options and care plans. Voice your preferences, concerns, and goals for treatment, and collaborate with your healthcare team to make informed decisions about your health. Ask about the risks, benefits, and alternatives to proposed treatments.

5. Advocate for Access to Care

Advocate for access to comprehensive, gender-sensitive healthcare services that address the unique needs of women with heart disease. Demand equitable access to preventive care, diagnostic testing, treatment options, and support services. Speak out against barriers to care such as financial constraints, geographic disparities, and lack of awareness.

Spreading Awareness and Education in the Community

1. Share Your Story

Share your personal experience with heart disease to raise awareness and educate others in your community. Speak at local events, support groups, or community forums about your journey with heart disease, the importance of early detection and prevention, and the challenges and triumphs of managing the condition.

2. Host Educational Workshops

Organize educational workshops or seminars focused on women's heart health in collaboration with local healthcare providers, community organizations, or advocacy groups. Cover topics such as risk factors, symptoms, prevention strategies, and treatment options, and provide resources and support for attendees.

3. Advocate for Policy Change

Advocate for policy change at the local, state, and national levels to improve access to preventive care, screening, and treatment for women with heart disease. Support initiatives that promote women's heart health awareness, research, education, and funding. Contact elected officials, participate in advocacy campaigns, and join advocacy organizations to amplify your voice.

4. Engage with Media and Social Media

Use traditional media outlets such as newspapers, radio, and television to raise awareness about women's heart health and share educational messages with a wider audience. Utilize social media platforms to share resources, articles, infographics, and personal stories about heart disease prevention and management, and encourage others to join the conversation.

5. Partner with Healthcare Providers and Organizations

Collaborate with healthcare providers, hospitals, clinics, and nonprofit organizations that specialize in women's heart health to expand outreach efforts and reach underserved communities. Participate in community health fairs, wellness events, and screenings to provide education, resources, and support to women in your community.

Empowering women to take charge of their heart health is essential for reducing the burden of heart disease and improving outcomes for women worldwide. By advocating for oneself in healthcare settings and spreading awareness and education in the community, women can make a meaningful impact on their own health and the health of others. Through education, engagement, and advocacy, women can prioritize their cardiovascular well-being and inspire positive change in their communities.

This comprehensive exploration of empowering women to take charge of their heart health provides readers with valuable strategies for advocating for themselves in healthcare settings and spreading awareness and education in the community. By taking a proactive approach to their health, engaging in shared decision making, and advocating for access to care, women can improve outcomes for themselves and others affected by heart disease. Through collaboration, education, and advocacy, women can empower themselves and their communities to prioritize cardiovascular health and well-being.

CHAPTER 12

The Future of Women's Heart Health

As we look ahead to the future of women's heart health, there is much optimism fueled by advances in research, treatment, and prevention strategies. In this chapter, we will explore the latest developments in the field, including promising research findings, innovative treatment modalities, and strategies for continued prevention and improvement of women's heart health.

Advances in Research and Treatment

1. Precision Medicine

Precision medicine holds great promise for personalized treatment approaches tailored to individual differences in genetics, lifestyle, and environment. By analyzing genetic markers and other biomarkers, researchers can identify subgroups of women at higher risk of heart disease and develop targeted interventions to improve outcomes.

2. Novel Therapies

Researchers are exploring novel therapeutic approaches for the treatment of heart disease in women, including gene therapy, stem cell therapy, and regenerative medicine. These innovative therapies aim to repair damaged heart tissue, restore cardiac function, and prevent disease progression, offering new hope for women with advanced cardiovascular conditions.

3. Pharmacogenomics

Pharmacogenomics is revolutionizing the way medications are prescribed and administered by considering individual genetic variations in drug response. By identifying genetic predictors of drug efficacy and adverse effects, researchers can optimize medication regimens for women with heart disease, maximizing benefits and minimizing risks.

4. Digital Health Technologies

Digital health technologies such as wearable devices, mobile apps, and telemedicine platforms are transforming the delivery of cardiovascular care for women. These technologies enable remote monitoring, real-time feedback, and personalized coaching, empowering women to actively manage their heart health and engage in preventive behaviors.

Strategies for Continued Prevention and Improvement

1. Gender-Specific Research

Increased funding and support for gender-specific research are essential for advancing our understanding of heart disease in women. By including more women in clinical trials and research studies, researchers can uncover sex-specific differences in disease mechanisms, risk factors, and treatment responses, leading to more effective interventions.

2. Early Detection and Prevention

Early detection and prevention remain key priorities for reducing the burden of heart disease in women. Public health initiatives aimed at raising awareness, promoting screening, and implementing preventive measures can help identify high-risk individuals and intervene early to prevent or delay the onset of heart disease.

3. Lifestyle Modification Programs

Comprehensive lifestyle modification programs that promote healthy eating, physical activity, stress management, and smoking cessation are essential for preventing and managing heart disease in women. These programs should be accessible, culturally tailored, and evidence-based to address the unique needs and preferences of diverse populations.

4. Multidisciplinary Care

Multidisciplinary care models that involve collaboration between primary care providers, cardiologists, nurses, dietitians, psychologists, and other healthcare professionals are crucial for delivering comprehensive and coordinated care to women with heart disease. These integrated care teams can address the complex biopsychosocial needs of women and improve outcomes.

5. Health Equity Initiatives

Addressing health disparities and promoting health equity are fundamental for ensuring that all women have access to high-quality cardiovascular care. Health equity initiatives should prioritize underserved populations, including racial and ethnic minorities, socioeconomically disadvantaged individuals, and rural communities, to reduce disparities in heart health outcomes.

Conclusion

The future of women's heart health is bright, with ongoing advances in research, treatment, and prevention strategies offering new hope for women worldwide. By harnessing the power of precision medicine, novel therapies, pharmacogenomics, and digital health technologies, researchers and healthcare providers can improve outcomes for women with heart disease and enhance their quality of life.

Through continued investment in gender-specific research, early detection and prevention efforts, lifestyle modification programs, multidisciplinary care models, and health equity initiatives, we can empower women to take control of their heart health and reduce the global burden of heart disease. By working together to implement innovative strategies and foster collaboration across disciplines, we can create a future where all women have the opportunity to live heart-healthy lives.

This comprehensive exploration of the future of women's heart health provides readers with valuable insights into advances in research, treatment, and prevention strategies. By embracing precision medicine, novel therapies, pharmacogenomics, and digital health technologies, researchers and healthcare providers can revolutionize the delivery of cardiovascular care for women. Through continued investment in gender-specific research, early detection and prevention efforts, lifestyle modification programs, multidisciplinary care models, and health equity initiatives, we can empower women to prioritize their cardiovascular well-being and improve outcomes for women with heart disease. Through collaboration, innovation, and advocacy, we can create a future where all women have the opportunity to thrive and live heart-healthy lives